CHALLENGE YOUR ENVIRONMENT

MARK RICHARDSON

Challenge your environment publishing

© 2012 MARK RICHARDSON

ISBN: 978-1985735149

DEDICATION

Challenge Your Environment's devoted to my beautiful family, but most of all, my wife, Josephine Richardson. Thank you for supporting me with your actions and not your words. When the mornings were cold and wet, you were right by my side rain or shine. When I was weak and wanted to go to the food dealer, you were my conscious after losing over 100 pounds; I now know that I can accomplish anything, even writing this book.

Table of CONTENTS

CHALLENGE YOUR ENVIRONMENT

MARK RICHARDSON

Life moves fast

Who is this writer, and why do I have his book in my hands? I'll tell you. In my opinion, I am nothing more than a typical red-blooded American, and like most Americans, I had a weight issue. I once weighed over three hundred plus pounds, and my equally sexy wife of twenty years plus years weighed in at two hundred and seventy pounds.

My wife and I fell in love on August 17, 1996. That was when I had the body of a young lifeguard with several weight-training classes, but that all changed rather quickly.

My wife and I became proud parents of three children by the time we were 24. Not only did we decided to have them young, we decided to have our two oldest boys 17 months apart. And un-school all three of them.

My wife volunteered to stay home with the children, which added to what I call the momma bear syndrome or weight gain for parents.
While my wife stayed home with the children, I put on papa bear weight by working upwards to three jobs doing whatever I could for income.

I worked any job I could get my hands on, which led to me working in many different fields, sometimes all at once. I worked as a bouncer, cashier, security officer for public schools, a School bus driver, truancy officer, and eventually a correctional officer/counselor for California's eighteen to twenty-five repeat felons in a medical, mental institution.

Naturally, I gained weight because I never stopped working out or even meditate on what I was doing. My weight issues only increased once I hit it big by becoming a correctional officer at the age of 22. After graduating from a 16-week academy, I worked as a prison guard schedule.

That means I now live in prison, and I visit my home. I live in a prison city, and I visit my family and the town I live in on my days off. I became a guest in my own home.

Stress Stores Fat

Money worries were over, but my stress level was about to take a big leap along with my waist size.

As they say, 'more money, more problems.' Once I started to make more money than I ever had before, my wife and I did what all young people in their 20's do - we spent it! We never thought about investing because we wanted to buy useless "things" and give our babies the best "stuff." The longer and harder the work shift, the more I justified terrible food. That intern made it harder, so I worked harder to lose weight.

I still had not learned about stress and how to manage it, so I pushed onward in my efforts to make more money.

By age twenty-four, I became a prison counselor at N.A Chaderjian for repeat drug sex, and murder inmates in a medical, mental lockup facility for eighteen to twenty-five repeat offenders, located in Stockton, California.

Being an employee in prison is terrible enough, let alone a medical, mental lock-up institution. You could imagine the wonders it did for my mind, gut, and butt. I was now regularly sitting and had become even more stressed out. I took on my counselor position when I weighed a whopping two hundred and fifty pounds to two hundred and sixty pounds.

After one and a half years of crazy 16 hour shifts and the 1-hour commute each way, I started to rack up weight and fast. I now weighed two hundred and eighteen pounds, and for a brief small Mila second, I touched over three hundred and fifteen pounds after only three years of the worst sleeping and eating habits of my life due to being a father of three and a Prison Guard/counselor.

I am like most Americans, as you can tell by now; I am no different from you. I, too, am a hard-working American that wants to enjoy his nights and weekends with good food friends and drinks. Humans are creatures of habit, so break your habits.

I realized that the change had to start in my head. I started the healing process by being 100% honest with myself in every aspect of my life.

Being honest with one's self is much harder to do than it sounds. At three hundred pounds, I felt like I was a skinny guy trapped in a fat man's body screaming for help, and nobody could hear or see me. Instead of giving up, I decided to fight and find my way out of this mess. After all, I put myself in this situation.

I had placed myself in a figurative prison cell, and I was the owner of the prison cell. That's when I realized that I had the keys to my prison cell. I needed to lose the weight on my own to free myself from myself.

We all make mistakes

I started my journey off as a typical American; I bought diet supplies. Gym clothes and water bottles to work out, and that lasted about one week. Once I fell off the physical exercise wagon, I stuck to my pills; I bought to help my diet and exercise.

That was a mistake. There is a reason the label says that the medicines best work with a balanced meal and exercise. Diet supplies imply that the change is going to be temporary and not a life change. Usually, the diet lasts as long as it is convenient. That leads me to the worst pills of my life.

I bought the most embarrassing diet pills of all time; they should have been illegal. The medicines act as a shock therapy type of treatment. If you eat greasy food, the drug will cause the grease from the diet to slip right out of your bum into your underwear or jeans. I had a very unfortunate misshape after eating a very greasy burger. Thank God, I had chosen to wear black pants that day. Let's say Pills are not the way to go. They are lazy and not a long term solution.

Stockholm's Syndrome and Your Fat

What is Stockholm's Syndrome? Stockholm's syndrome or capture-bonding is a psychological phenomenon in which hostages express empathy and sympathy and have positive feelings toward their captors, sometimes to the point of defending and identifying with them. You know that you have heard the excuses made by comedians and your friends that "You have to love yourself no matter how big you get."

To some extent, they are correct. You have to love yourself enough to see that you are the cause of your imprisonment, and you like yourself enough to get out of your self-imposed confinement. You have to change your perception of your situation to improve your reality.

If you are overweight and you have no illness that causes the weight gain, you need to recognize that you are the cause of your fat imprisonment and possible diseases.

To remove yourself from the prison of obesity, you must first recognize that you put yourself into the cell to hide, escape, or protect yourself from something in your life. You may be hiding from child abuse, neglect, coming from poverty, or like most Americans, unchecked drug addiction to food. Food is a socially acceptable drug, which is why it is up to you to free ourselves.

We must challenge our environment around us. We are unique individuals with unique individuals surrounding us at any given time. Some of these exceptional people we allow around us help us justify making the wrong choices. However, in life, we must recognize our power to control ourselves and our ability to give our power to others to control us.

We justify our actions by allowing our friends to decide on what we eat or do for pleasure. By doing so, we give ourselves an out or excuse from being fully responsible for our actions.

I remember a quote from the prison, "To not make a decision is to have made a decision not to make a decision. Your choice was not to make one or not to cast your vote as it is said.

Once you realize that you are your captor, the next steps are up to you. All that you are required to do is to reach down into your pocket, remove the keys that open the prison cell door, and free yourself. Stop screaming from behind the door to someone that is not there.

Stop telling the figment of your imagination that you want out of the cell when you are the person that put you in your prison cell, to begin. What is making you so unhappy that you cannot gather the strength to pull yourself up and say no to excess food, T.V, excessive drinking, and other bad habits we adapt to our lives? The power is indeed in your hands.

you are reading this book or any other book on weight loss; you are trying to break free from the hold of your captor "Fat." That is the start. There is no way to break out of your bonds and set yourself free if you do not search for a way out of them. We do not just figuratively lock ourselves up; we do it too. How many times have you refused to do an activity because of your weight?

How many times have you been too tired from sitting all day, so you turn down the walk around the park with a friend?

Maybe you're like my wife; she was to get off the roller coaster ride, due to her weight and her inability to buckle her seat belt. Her weight that day controlled her happiness. In California, a famous restaurant was closed and forced to relocate. Someone was too overweight to fit through the doors of the restaurant Squeez inn Burger.

Instead of seeing what they had done to themselves by eating that kind of food, she tried to sue the burger shop and have them closed down. The business just moved to a new location and found a way to keep their livelihood going.

The person that tried to sue them was obese and is a clear case of a person controlled by their captor. Her addiction convinced her that these people were not thoughtful by not make room for her and her excessive weight. And this is where the dependence or "Food" becomes acceptable. You have one group that will say we are discriminating against her by not providing chairs strong enough to hold her and another that sues because the doors are not wide enough.

If a person knowingly causes harm to himself or herself, it is labeled self-abuse.

The burger shack individual felt that they should be able to enjoy the same foods and life as an active person. Reality check! You cannot! The burger check person was and still is in a figurative prison. The worst part about this prison is that you are the only one that is keeping you in it. We have the keys to our cell and the prison door; you have to want freedom more than that burger or any addiction for that matter.

You have to want to take control of your life and set yourself free. Challenge your environment! Never give up! Never surrender!
Try this small experiment, if you are twenty-five pounds overweight, get a twenty-five pound dumbbell, and Start walking around the gym for 3 hours with the weight.

What you'll get is a taste of what your Heart, Back, Legs, and Torso are feeling, except your heart never puts the weights down.
Now try to lie to yourself and tell yourself that those 25 pounds you walked around with were not very heavy or much weight on your heart.

Your heart is the motor of your body. You should never carry long-term excess weight. So, if you can walk around with the dumbbells literally in your hands, do not make your heart move that and more. The thing about weight loss is that it is 100% all on you.

If you choose liposuction, pills, shakes, personal trainers, Px90, or any other form of weight loss, you have to make the appointment, pay for the supplies, go to the doctor, or go to the store to purchase these things. You have to get up and apply the effort to gain the results you want to experience.

The point I am trying to drive home is that it takes action, no matter what route you choose. Decisive reactions in the right step can and will help everybody get a step closer to being free from their captor. One of the most freeing actions you can take is lacing your shoes up and walking every day for twenty minutes and drink as much water as possible, if not exclusively.

By starting with small steps, you begin to take steps towards excessive weight loss, but you must start today. Do not put off until tomorrow what you can accomplish today!

Baby steps are the best for any overweight person. We spent most of our time watching T.V shows. If we were not cooking the food, we were watching the grub on T.V. If we are not preparing it for ourselves, we are making it for our friends and families that expect. These are the same people that hope you have food or sweets in your house. It takes baby steps for everyone around you to get used to your new way of life

My diet

I tried everything. I tried pills that block your body from absorbing the fat from the food you eat so that you do not have to stop being a fat glutinous pig. That is right. You read it right; you can still taste nasty, kill you, pickle your liver fast food, and even lose weight. And the diet pill was right to a degree, and it's what I call the 'shock treatment diet.'

The best way for me to explain this pill to you is by Dawn soap. Yes, "Dawn soap the stuff that sticks to the grease on the pots and cleans your dishes."

Do you know how it makes the grease run away when you put a drop in your dirty pots?

Well, these pills work similarly. When you eat a big fat juicy grease burger, you take that little pill, and it stops your body from absorbing the grease, which now allows the oil to slip right out the back door, no matter what you want.

What you end up with is an orange or grease color in your underwear, if you are lucky.

If you are not lucky, you will absorb more grease then your body can hold onto, and the next thing you know, you are slipping out of your chair and your pants, because it is grease sliding out of your bum! What can your sphincter muscles do against oil?

Then you have the diets that have you eat nothing but meat. Not good! That is how you ended up with the worst poo and scared up toilets. Your body is not designed to eat so much meat. Think about it!

We're a part of the food chain.

Some point and time in history we had a meeting and decided that as the human race we are above nature and we can eat the way we want, as much as we want, and then get mad that we don't look as sleek and as strong as the lion that eats enormous portions of meat.

One significant fact is that we, as super-intelligent humans did not take into account is that Lions weighs somewhere around 600 to 800 pounds.

A lion can go up to 4 days without eating, after a good kill.

We usually sit in an air-conditioned office and drive ourselves in oversized vehicles everywhere. Still, somehow we get the feeling that we need as much meat as possible on a daily bases.

Why?

Because you have to Challenge your environment to get your mind right to lose weight, before you can drop any real fat and keep it off, you will have to put your Brain in a place that will allow it to accept your new way of life. You will have to change the way you see things in your life.

Your perception is going to have to change for your reality to change.

I first stumbled on the solution to my weight problem, about two hundred and eighty-eight pounds, and seven years on the job in prison. I realized I had to gain a positive perception of everything in my life.

As usual, I was working an overtime shift (not by choice) just finishing some case notes on one of the inmates assigned to me when out of nowhere, I started thinking about him and his drug addiction. His addiction was no different from my addiction to the big fat juicy steak burrito that I was about to devour, accept my addiction was sold on the side of the road, and is socially acceptable.

Now, some might think, 'what's wrong with that? Man's got to eat?' Well, here is the problem. I bought two of those massive burritos we all know and love, but I was only four hours into my shift when I reached for my second burrito.

My food addiction was so severe I could not even make it the two-mile distance from the burrito truck to my job before I had already torn into the first one.

My drug of choice is food

I was unable to control my desire for food, and I was now what society lovingly calls a "Crack Head" but not for crack. I had it for something that I could get any time day or night. I even had it delivered to me. I was officially a "Food head." To gain control of my life, I decided to apply the lessons that I had been teaching the inmates with a drug addiction issue.

First, I had to acknowledge the fact that I was no better than the last individual that was recently in my office. I had my very own addiction, but my obsession is not to a big evil publicly hated drug dealer; it was to food. All different sorts of food!

Starting my recovery

Anything I saw I wanted, and with the job I had, I could buy and eat any food I wanted anytime I wanted. That should be that I had a significant lack of self-control, and that was going to be a challenge I was going to have to overcome.

The first thing I did was admit to myself, "I had a problem." At that moment, I looked down at my massive gut and my roach coach burrito sitting on my desk and realized I had been lying to myself.

Next, I put the food away and walked out of the room. I set an alarm clock so that I could eat when it was supposed to. I figured I went to public school; I was programmed to eat at a scheduled time, and I need to get back into that routine.

It was easier than I thought to fall back into that routine, only this time I was going to be in control. I figured that if an individual chose to control themselves sexually, emotionally, one could also deprive himself of what he truly wants. So I made sure to deprive myself of things I knew I did not need, and in return, I proved to myself that I had self-control and the power to set myself free from the prison I trapped myself in.

I learned to talk to myself and ask myself the same question I asked the inmates assigned to my caseload.

"Are you being honest with yourself? Was that answer to the previous question, the truth? With a quick follow up, "Are you aware you're your response doesn't matter unless you're honest with yourself?

Finally, I followed up with, "Once you enter your cell, you will either be alone with an honest person or a liar.

That was all the reminder I needed to whip myself back into shape as they say. I've never liked it when a doctor would tell me I need to lose weight or I'm going to die. Meanwhile, he reeks of cigarettes. On the other hand, you have the guy that tells you how to lose weight but has never been overweight in their life, so what do they know of the body pains and heartache that we go through.

Essentially, what I am saying is we as humans naturally prefer to take advice from people that are a real live example of what they believe.

If you can be completely honest with yourself, your actions will show everybody that you told yourself the truth. If you cannot be honest with yourself, then you are just living a lie, and a lie is no way to live.

So I promised myself that I wouldn't talk about anything to anybody I just needed to make changes. By doing that, everybody around me will see how serious I am about my life.

If you have an overweight belly and you know that you're eating way too much food, too much of the wrong food or not working out nearly enough, ask yourself, "Do I deserve the big fat juicy burrito, burger or steak tonight?" Does my body indeed need this, or is this a lack of self-control.

Working 16 hours a day, commuting two hours round trip and no actual exercise was killing me. I was taking in more calories than I was using daily. I wasn't working on a construction site like I did when I was eighteen in my father's business.
I was behaving like most Americans — eating and not working out.

I had to change the way I looked at food and fast or how I looked at fast food. One method that helped me challenge my environment and win consistently was writing down what I had in my environment. Write in a food journal. Keep track of how you feel as you begin your journey. Write notes about your sleeping habits and bathroom habits.

Your notes will act as a visual representation of what your hour, day, week, or moth honestly looks like, it will also help you see how much time or how many "Man-hours" you've devoted to your heart, lungs, mind, or muscles.

I came up with "Man-hours" while working with high school students. I watched these kids that barely even knew each other swap so much body fluid in the middle of the hallways that hazmat suits had to be used to separate them.

The amount of time they spent getting to know the individual they were sucking face with was not even enough time to get a twenty-cent raise on a job. Most jobs require at least a six-month minimum before they also talk to you about a long-term commitment. So ask yourself, "how many Man-hours do you dedicate to your health? Honestly, ask yourself if you are eating to live or living to eat. Keep a food journal.

It is a way to help you track all of the foods or the amounts of calories you're either putting into your body. You will be able to see what you ate burning vs. storing. Track how many "Man-hours" you are dedicating to T.V versus walking or doing something proactive in your weight loss. Use part of this page to write the thought that comes to you when you are reading this. There is no time like the present to start making the necessary changes needed to reach your health goals.

When it comes to losing weight, the fight can only be fought by you and you alone. You hold the keys to your prison cell. The ability to start and stop your progress is entirely up to you and no one else.

Your body is like a car

Your perception controls your reality, and your reality is a significant part of weight loss. How you perceive things in your environment decided on how you will interact with your environment. So to use that to your advantage, view yourself as a car. A fuel gulping gas spewing pollutant that needs to be taken to the shop to be kept in good condition.

"If you have a full tank of gas and don't need to fill up, so you don't stop to spend an over-inflated amount of money on gas for you don't. Like a car, your extra fuel will overflow onto the ground or over your beltline, causing a possible explosion. Tell yourself that you'll fuel up when you get to your side of town, where you know the gas is better for your car and cheaper on your pocketbook."

The key is being honest with yourself, and knowing when to say enough is something only you can tell. Recognize the difference in eating Just because you can, and ask yourself if you should. You can put your hand in the fire, but should you. It may sound like I am saying starve yourself, but that is precisely not what I am saying.

I am merely saying that if you have not exerted the amount of energy that you have eaten for the day, you are storing energy away in fat cells. Stored energy is merely fat that you have not converted into energy.

As we all know, fat's for hard times, so ask yourself, when are you going to have a hard time? When will food a food shortage if there is a form of food on every corner in most Westernized countries? If you're honest, your answers should be "never! That means it will take you to be honest with yourself if you want to change your life in any way. You have to tell yourself the truth - I am overweight, and I want to change it. If you genuinely want to change, it will come from inside.

Only you control you and what goes in or out of your mouth. You have to read the ingredients and know what you are eating. Then, be honest with yourself and ask yourself if you should eat it?

Do not use justification for breaking your own rules. If you made a rule to only eat vegetables that day, don't give in just because your coworker brings in   The more you resist and conquer the junk food demons, the more make the mental changes needed, the more you will see the physical changes you want.

T.V is the enemy

You're Visual Sensors React to Commercials!
I know you've heard this for years, but it's very accurate. According to a report written by Ingrid Lunden, a reporter for TechCrunch comes from paidContent.org, where she was a staff writer and has also written freelance articles for other publications such as the Financial Times. Ingrid covers mobile, digital media, advertising, and the spaces where these intersect.

According to Ingrid Lunden's research, it indicates that although women spend almost forty minutes more than men watching straight television every day — four hours, eleven minutes for women; three hours thirty-four minutes for men — men are spending more than twice as much time as women using gaming consoles — plainly forty-eight minutes compared to twenty-two minutes each day.

Add that usage to TV time and the gap between how much time men and women spend in front of the screen narrows — although women are still ahead of men in TV screen time by a space of 11 minutes.
If you're to change your perception of the T.V. and see it as a short Cyclops, that's only here to suck your time and thoughts away.

How can you be thinking when you're watching, monitoring, and feeling emotional connections with a T.V?

As for those that think you're thinking with the T.V on, wait until you see what you can do a few weeks after the crack/time-waster is no longer controlling your mind. When you take time from the T.V, you will find that T.V. keeps you in a state of excitement or drama and too much of anything is bad for you.

One way to tell if T.V is consuming your life is to see what your day to day thoughts and topics are when you're at work.

Do your thoughts consist of T.V questions such as, 'Will they get off the island,' will finally get married?' Who cares? First, you have to ask why you should even care about what the in shape, hot, and sexy actors are doing at work. Don't forget that being hot and sexy on T.V is what they get paid to do. Focus on yourself and how you can become hot and sexy.

Actors have the luxury of being on the beach, creating their shows or movies. They can afford a personal trainer to keep them on task, while you gain pound after pound and New Year's resolution after New Year's resolution. How do you feel about continuing your life on the couch while the T.V Cyclops sucks your youth, time, thoughts, and energy away, just so that you can find out who is having sex with who and who was spotted where doing god knows what!

You need to be the sexy person getting spotted in wild places by your associates while you're in shape because you were able to get your mind right to shake the weight off.

When an actor needs to be motivated, they can afford to get a personal trainer to come to their house and push them. They also have their enormous paychecks that we provide by staying fat and devoting more time to T.V. than to our very own lives.

You have to change the way you see your time. How much time do you spend in the sun with sweat building up on your skin, causing goosebumps to form and run down your spine? I found walking to be my number one way of losing weight. It was much more comfortable to walk than it was to jog at 300 pounds.

<u>*After my weight started to shake Off*</u>

At this point and time of my life, I was honest with myself about all of the foods I put in my mouth and home. I kept focused on the fact that you are a product of your environment, so I made sure to keep my environment a healthy one.

By creating a clean, healthy space in my home, it helped keep my mind fresh and health. It made it easier for me to drop pounds fast, so fast that I felt like I need to go to the doctor to make sure I wasn't sick. After all, I worked in a medical, mental prison. As a counselor, I spent lots of time with people that have different types of severe illnesses that are highly contagious.

It was just one of the many dangers to the job, along with being attacked killed or having my family stocked by an angry parolee.

But to my relief, I was losing a large amount of weight from my life change. I cut out T.V. entirely for eight months. I still ate fast food, so to say I didn't eat the most addictive drug on the planet would be a lie and hypocritical. I ate just the burger from the fast-food chains. But then the time came when I had to have another heart to heart with myself again and this time get even more honest with me. I had to stop eating the garbage altogether. I promised myself that I would only eat homemade food and fresh fruits and vegetables.

After the "Let's stop lying to myself," the talk I gave myself over and over again," I decided it was time to get myself educated on how to stay in shape. I wanted to remain equipped with enough knowledge to battle the cravings that the smell of fast food brings to me. I had to be armed and ready to fight those feelings of happiness that come with giving into my addiction.

I started building my armory of weapons by not watching but studying one of the documentaries called "Fast Food Nation" and "Supersize Me." After that, I made a short journey down the road to Food Matters, while stopping off for the occasional episode of You Are What You Eat.

These were shows that kept me focused on not slipping back into bad habits. By staying focused on being honest with what I want for my life, I now fit into clothes I didn't know existed.
That was motivation enough!

One day I wanted to show my wife just how much weight I lost. I put on her pants, and I showed her that I had lots of room in her pants.

I have to say that that was the moment that made my wife sit down in front of the mirror and have the one on one she needed with herself.

My wife found as I did that when she placed herself in front of the mirror, she noticed in her reflection that she had her soda in her hand as usual. It hit her that Soda was her drug of choice, her crack if you will. It was the exact moment she realized that she was killing herself just like her father was.

He was an alcoholic. He died at a very young age. Believe me, if you get your mind right and you are truly honest with yourself, you, too, can look like the hot and sexy time stealing actors.

Look at the time in what I like to call your estimated life span. We hope that we can live happy seventy to ninety years. But in those seventy to ninety years, how much would it hurt you, if for the next six months or even six years of your remaining time you eat healthily? What if you only took six months out of your life to drink water? What would be the worst-case scenario if you promised your body that you were not going to eat grease, fat, fake food, or unhealthy high fructose corn syrup for my source of energy?

If you take six months, you will find that you have plenty of time to fall off the wagon and go back to your old ways. You can then do whatever it is that you want to do to your body. I have to say, after being in great form to being out of shape to being back in my correct figure, "There is nothing sweeter than being thin." If you look at your day-to-day and your week-to-week with the intent to make time, you will find that you have become devoted to things that could be replaced or moved around.

It is wise to try and dedicate about six months to you and your mind. You cannot fix the body if you do not adjust your brain. Time is never-ending; you can't control it, learn to manage it. What I mean by that is there will always be something there to take up your time, but it is up to you to put things in priority of what needs to come first.

Your health or the late-night runs to the local pub or fast food joint? Use that time for just six months out of your seventy to ninety-year life span to do some pushups, watch a documentary that will remind you why you don't eat that way, read a book, or write down the reasons why you think you put on so much weight. You have to learn to talk to yourself and ask real questions that only you know the answers too. The time you spend for six months just walking and thinking and talking with a partner or friend will feel like the life you're living is so much better than the old one that you won't want to go back too. I promise.

You will also find that by being knockdown, drag-out honest with yourself, there were a lot more things causing your weight gain than just T.V.

Monster Work Out

This portion of the book is perfect for everyone but is focused more on the parents than the none parents.

My exercise once the T.V. went off.

I realized my 11, 9, and 7-year-olds were bored out of their minds, so I decided to give them a taste of my childhood. We went to the local park, and I became the monster that had to chase the children and devour them. They loved it. It not only gave me more endurance to play with my kids, but it also gave me more energy in the bedroom to chase my wife down.

I would climb up the ladder on the jungle gym and run across the bridge, then slide down the firemen's pole. It was exhausting work.

The children understood daddy needed a few breaks to keep up the effort I was putting out. The laughter of my children drove me to want to work harder, so I will be able to hike and run after my grandkids someday. I remember asking my wife, "How long do you think you could run after the guy who takes your kid?" We both thought about it and realized we needed to change. But we didn't. I was two hundred and eighty-eight pounds.

 I pose the question to you. How long do you think you would be able to run if your child's taken from you?

What is exercise? One dictionary gave me these answers.

•	An act of employing or putting into play; use: the free exercise of intellect; the exercise of an option.

•	An activity that requires physical or mental exertion, primarily when performed to develop or maintain fitness: took an hour of vigorous daily exercise at a gym.

A task, problem, or other effort performed to develop or maintain fitness or increase skill: a piano exercise; a memory exercise.

You can see how exercising your mind and body is needed to stay balanced.

You have to make your mind remember your goals and expectations. You can't let it tell your body, 'I can rest today.' Not if you know that you have not earned the rest. Be honest with yourself. It is exhausting but worth it.

How horrible would it be if what stood between you and your child's safety was a large gut caused by a few cheeseburgers or tacos? If someone snatched your child in front of you at the park, could you run long enough to apprehend the kidnapper, or would they getaway? Could you run fast enough, hard enough, and long enough to catch the criminal?

It only takes thirty-minutes a day to build a long-lasting relationship with your kids at the park, and you gain physical endurance. Never mind that you are teaching them to take their health seriously, and you are teaching them how to be an excellent interactive parent for the future when they become worn out exhausted parents.

The more you play, the more your body gets used to running and jumping. Your brain loves oxygen, and your actions will build excellent muscle memory. One plus is your children are always up for a day, or even an hour, at the park.

Crazy Apples

I titled this chapter Crazy Apples because this is one of my favorite workouts. I eat an apple or two for breakfast, then put on my favorite jams and just let loose.

Now, be very honest with yourself - are you dancing as hard as you could, or are you embarrassed by what people think of you, even yourself? I would put on my absolute favorite music and lose it. I looked like Kevin Bacon from the movie Footloose. What I found was that I was losing weight just because I was moving my body.

I was not only letting my energy stay stored in my stomach and legs; I was using it. All of the fruits and vegetables I had been eating acted like high-octane gas in my tank. It made me want to keep eating fruits and vegetables throughout the day and, of course, other things like peanut butter and honey on wheat.

I did this workout in the morning about four times a week (you need some time to rest).

When you work out, you're using the stored energy in fat cells. If you stop and do five to ten pushups three times a day, you will see a significant difference in your chest, arms, and back after about two weeks.

So, after six months of just dancing to your favorite music and cutting out the extra fat in your life, you will lose lots of weight.

Write down your food plan for each day on a page, use this for the first time.

1.

2.

3.

4.

5.

6.

7.

8.

9.

10.

11.

12.

13.

14.

15.

16.

17.

18.

20.

21.

22.

23.

24.

25.

26.

27.

28.

29.

30.

31.

MARK RICHARDSON

Eat breakfast

Believe it or not, eating breakfast is better than not eating breakfast at all. Some breakfast options are better than others. Getting the right combination of nutrients will help you feel full of energy and just plain full until lunch, while eating the wrong foods for breakfast may have you reaching for a doughnut or other less healthy snack option a short time later.

One of the key components to weight loss is fresh fruit combined with a healthy breakfast that they provide vitamins, minerals, water, and fiber. Fiber helps to slow down the digestive process and keep you full longer. The vitamins and minerals help you meet your daily requirements for these nutrients, which is hard to do if you skip breakfast.

Oatmeal with fruit and milk, yogurt with
fruit and granola, a fruit smoothie with toast and peanut butter, and fruit juice with a breakfast burrito made with a whole grain tortilla all make delicious and nutritious options for breakfast.

You can stock up on portable breakfast options to make it easier to fit this meal into your days, such as fruits that are easy to carry with you, granola bars, and cups of yogurt.

Crazy Apples is more than just apples; it is about all kinds of fruits that get you moving and staying moving.

The goal is to put on your favorite song and move for as long as you can. Since the beginning of time, humans and music have gone hand in hand.

Music takes your mind off physical pain, sorrow,   and time. You can listen to a whole CD and not realize you just spent two hours listing to your favorite jam, and the most you did was bob your head. If you love it, dance, move, burn fat, and feel tired.

The more you move, the more you burn. The more excitement you have and use towards dancing, the more heat you generate heat. The more energy you exert, the smaller your pant or dress size will get. Its simple math. Eat less lousy food and work out more. The other fantastic quality about Crazy Apples is that if you do have a physically active job, you will add more cardio to your daily workout. That, in turn, means you will burn twice as much fat in one day. The more you scorch, the more fat gets transformed from storage into energy for your mind and body. Soon you will be losing lots and lots of fat all over your body.

You will notice that your neck has shrunk, reunited with your feet, and other parts that have gone missing, reappear.

Do not go over your max for the day.

That is what I call a surplus. You have saved enough space to put some fat back into the bank. Feel free to have that nice dinner at the restaurant and the extra drink that day. But be sure to take it day by day, not week by week. After all, yesterday and tomorrow do n't exist, only now does. So if you mess up, it is ok. Just fix it immediately and don't wait until tomorrow because tomorrow doesn't exist. Fruits and vegetables are a vital source of vitamins, minerals, and fiber that support a healthy body and prevent serious illnesses.

A diet rich in fruits and vegetables helps us maintain healthy, happy well-being, and it also is the first fighter in helping the body combat stress.

Water for 6 Months

It is only six months out of your entire 80-year life span. Really, how much is that? All I am asking is that you suck down water for six months to see how your body reacts to it. Your skin will clear up, your body will thank you with better bowel movements, and your organs will plain feel better.

The modification will only take a few months out of your 90-year life span. What is stopping you from devoting a little bit of time to your body's wellbeing? We have no problem with eating spicy stuff when we shouldn't or drinking too many nights in a row.

We will ask so much from our body but give it so little. We think we are giving it good stuff, but do you take it for a walk like your dog needs?

Do you feed it right like your dog is supposed to be feed?

Do you treat other's lives better than your own life? Pretend your mind is separate from your body. Your brain may sleep great, you may be smart as a whip, but if your brain's kicked, slapped, and abused, it will die. So your body will die, but your mind will feel firm.

The computer will function, but without its shell to protect it from destructive particles, it will die, and so will your brain. Water is the most important thing your body can have. It cleans all your organs, along with the largest one of all, your skin. You sweat all the time when you work out and drink water.

Water is undoubtedly an essential substance and the most abundant substance in the human body. Water comprises about three-quarters of the human mass and is a significant component of every cell.

Water is also vital for removing toxins from the human body.

The body removes toxins in many ways bowels, urination, and sweat. These methods directly excrete water from the body. When dehydrated, our bodies will try to save water by minimizing the use of the first three functions and will force the liver to assume as much of the workload as possible.
 This extra work will place a heavy burden on the liver, which has other functions in addition to detoxification. Even then, the liver by itself will not be able to do all the work very efficiently, and toxins will build up rapidly.

Water is also crucial to fitness and fat loss for several reasons, including the following: Water fills us up without adding any calories.

Dehydration will degrade a person's ability to exercise and burn calories. Dehydration will reduce protein synthesis, which is needed to build and repair muscles. The average persons recommended drinking about two to three quarts of water per day, however. The amount of water individual drinks will vary with the size and activity level of the person, as well as with climate conditions. Either case, if your urine is bright yellow, then you need to drink more water.

Also, anyone who exercises nonstop for more than an hour should consider replacing electrolytes along with the water. Drink electrolytes to avoid hypernatremia (depleted sodium) or other forms of severe electrolyte depletion, which can be dangerous.

Water is so essential that without it

YOU WILL DIE!

MARK RICHARDSON

A way of Life Change

This chapter is; "A Way of Life Change" because a diet is something you do when you want to fit into something for a weekend, not something you do for life. You have to make changes that will come over time. They will become part of your everyday routine, and your friends will even learn to accept whatever habit you have to keep you healthy and in shape.

Your spouse will encourage your workout, and your friends will either be jealous or support you. No matter what happens, you have to find joy in working out and in yourself.
Changing your life has to be something you enjoy for this to become a part of your life. It is why it is so crucial for you to change your perception so that your perception will change your reality.

By doing these things, you can get your mind right and not just accomplish weight loss but anything.

Once you make whatever routine that works for your work, you will feel powerful enough to take on the world. After all, anyone who can fight the fat demon and win will defiantly feel ready for any battle in their life. You must find something that works.

There are too many forms of exercise, such as walking, running, jogging, swimming, hiking, canoeing, kayaking, dancing, weight lifting, bike riding, rock climbing, and many, many more. That was just off the top of my head. You have to think, was there anything you liked doing when you were a kid that could make you lose weight. My wife took fencing classes.

That takes more skill and muscle control than one would ever think.
Try out something new. Losing weight is about more than fitting in clothes and being liked by the people around you. Even when you are not fat anymore, they will find another reason to dislike you, so you have to want to change for you for at least six months out of your life, but start now.

Nothing is stopping you from feeling like me except yourself. Break free of the prison you have placed yourself in and become more powerful than you have ever felt before. I've had my weight off for seven years now, and I am working on my sculpting.

Make a life change by getting your mind right. The rest will follow. After all, the body only goes where the head allows it to go. And now, the conclusion of my book, where you put down the book and decide, do I continue down the path of obesity and body odors, or do I start making changes? You have to decide if this book was worth your time.
The only way to show it was worth your time is through your actions, so get up, put on your shoes, and start the first of many new days in your new life. You and only you have the power to change you!

If you noticed, this book is somewhat short, and the reason for that is because you need to spend your time walking and exercising, not reading a novel on how to lose weight.

LACE YOUR SHOES UP AND START WALKING!

ABOUT THE AUTHOR

I was born in Sacramento, California, in 1979. I married my high school sweetheart and started supporting my family at age 19 by becoming a school bus driver. Two years later, I took on a new position for the school district supervising seven schools. I assisted the principals by keeping the school up to date on the local gang's graffiti and truancy/after school fights.

Two years later, I took on the department of corrections medical, mental institution by 22.